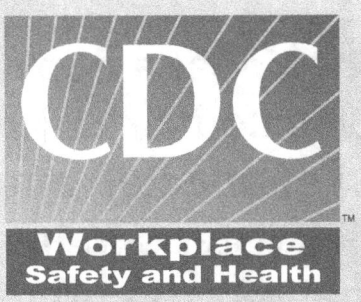

Evaluation of Cancer among Occupants of Two Office Buildings

Elena Page, MD, MPH

Gregory Burr, CIH

Scott Brueck, MS, CIH

Health Hazard Evaluation Report
HETA 2008-0166-3079
NASA Glenn Research Center
Cleveland, Ohio
March 2009

DEPARTMENT OF HEALTH AND HUMAN SERVICES
Centers for Disease Control and Prevention

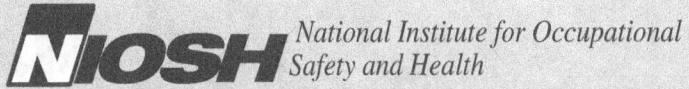 National Institute for Occupational Safety and Health

The employer shall post a copy of this report for a period of 30 calendar days at or near the workplace(s) of affected employees. The employer shall take steps to insure that the posted determinations are not altered, defaced, or covered by other material during such period. [37 FR 23640, November 7, 1972, as amended at 45 FR 2653, January 14, 1980].

CONTENTS

REPORT

Abbreviations ii

Highlights of the NIOSH Health Hazard Evaluation iii

Summary v

Introduction 1

Assessment 2

Results 3

Discussion 5

Conclusions 12

Recommendations 12

References 13

ACKNOWLEDGMENTS   Acknowledgments and Availability of Report 19

ABBREVIATIONS

ASHRAE	American Society of Heating, Refrigerating, and Air-Conditioning Engineers
GRC	Glenn Research Center
HEPA	High-efficiency particulate air
HHE	Health hazard evaluation
IEQ	Indoor environmental quality
HVAC	Heating, ventilating, and air conditioning
LESA	Lewis Engineers and Scientists Association
NAICS	North American Industry Classification System
NIOSH	National Institute for Occupational Safety and Health
NASA	National Aeronautics and Space Administration

The National Institute for Occupational Safety and Health (NIOSH) received a management request for a health hazard evaluation (HHE) at the National Aeronautics and Space Administration Glenn Research Center (GRC) in Cleveland, Ohio. The request was about ongoing employee and union concerns about a possible higher rate of cancer among current and former employees of Buildings 500 and 501. A site visit was made in October 2008.

What NIOSH Did

- We looked at asbestos reports and environmental sampling from the past 14 years from Buildings 500 and 501. We also looked at responses to concerns from building occupants.

- We reviewed surveys from current and former employees in Buildings 500 and 501. Some survey respondents had cancer. These surveys were provided by individual employees, management, and the union (Lewis Engineers and Scientists Association).

- We reviewed a confidential list of employees who have cancer. This list was provided by a supervisor.

- We looked at a list of retirements, medical and regular, from both buildings for the past 5 years. This list was provided by the GRC human resources office.

- We surveyed Buildings 500 and 501 to evaluate indoor environmental quality (IEQ) and the ventilation systems. We also measured carbon dioxide, temperature, and relative humidity.

- We checked facility records for evidence of previous environmental contamination of the air or drinking water.

What NIOSH Found

- Twenty different types of cancer were diagnosed among employees of Buildings 500 and 501.

- The most common types of cancer diagnosed were breast, lung, and prostate. These are the three most common cancers in the United States.

- The different types of cancers do not suggest a common exposure among employees diagnosed with cancer.

- The number of cancer cases and types of cancers do not appear unusual.

- No significant hazardous exposures were found in or near the two buildings.

- On the day of this evaluation, the carbon dioxide, temperature, and relative humidity levels in both buildings were within acceptable IEQ guidelines.

- Much of the asbestos in Buildings 500 and 501 had been removed, and the remaining was being correctly managed in place.

HIGHLIGHTS OF THE NIOSH HEALTH HAZARD EVALUATION (CONTINUED)

- Minor IEQ problems were found, such as water damage and poorly maintained fan coil units. These problems are not associated with the cancers diagnosed among employees.

What NIOSH Recommends

- No further investigation into the reported cancers is recommended.

- Management and union officials should encourage employees to learn about known cancer risk factors, measures they can take to reduce their risk for preventable cancers, and availability of cancer screening programs for certain types of cancer.

- Improve maintenance of fan coil units.

SUMMARY

NIOSH investigators evaluated employee and union concerns about a possible higher rate of cancer among current and former employees of Buildings 500 and 501. We found no hazardous exposures in these buildings. The types of cancers were not unusual, and the different types of cancers did not suggest a common exposure. We recommend no further investigation into the cancers reported in these buildings, but do encourage employees to learn about cancer risk factors, ways to reduce the risk for preventable cancers, and availability of cancer screening programs for certain types of cancer.

On October 11, 2007, NIOSH received a request for an HHE from the management of the NASA GRC in Cleveland, Ohio, regarding ongoing employee and union concerns about a possible higher rate of cancer among current and former employees of Buildings 500 and 501. This was the second HHE request NIOSH had received regarding this issue. The first request, received in 2004, was also submitted by management. In response to the first request, NIOSH investigators identified no hazardous exposures and closed the HHE with a letter [NIOSH 2004]. In this latest request, NASA GRC management explained that cancer concerns had resurfaced, no cause for these cancers had been identified, and employees were concerned about potential exposure to jet fuel and deicing compounds from the nearby airport, asbestos in the buildings, water damage in the buildings, and general IEQ.

This evaluation focused on the employees in Buildings 500 and 501, adjacent three-story brick office buildings constructed in the early 1960s. Building 500 has approximately 110,000 square feet of office space, and Building 501 has about 25,000 square feet; neither building has research labs. Both buildings are on the NASA GRC campus and across the road from the Cleveland Hopkins International Airport. We reviewed reports provided by NASA GRC management concerning asbestos remediation in these buildings, responses to complaints from building occupants, and environmental sampling during the past 14 years. We evaluated surveys about cancer diagnoses from current and former employees in Buildings 500 and 501 that were provided to us by LESA and NASA management. Additionally, a supervisor sent a confidential list of employees with cancer, and the NASA GRC human resources office provided a list of medical and regular retirements from the buildings during the past 5 years. We spoke with representatives from the Ohio Environmental Protection Agency regarding any past or current environmental contamination issues involving Buildings 500 and 501. We also consulted with representatives from the Ohio Department of Health's cancer registry.

We visited the site on October 7–8, 2008. On October 7, 2008, we held an opening meeting with representatives of management and LESA, then walked through the buildings, took measurements of IEQ comfort parameters, and looked for evidence of water damage, water incursion, visible mold, and other potential IEQ problems. On October 8, 2008, we gave two presentations to employees regarding the findings of our evaluation of the cancers

SUMMARY
(CONTINUED)

reported among employees, and then had a closing conference with representatives of management and LESA.

Twenty different types of cancer were diagnosed among employees of Buildings 500 and 501 since 1985. The most common types of cancer diagnosed were breast (17 cases), lung (7 cases), and prostate (4 cases), which are the three most common cancers in the United States. The other types of cancer diagnosed were melanoma, nonmelanoma skin cancer, colon, thyroid, bladder, pancreatic, cervical, uterine, head and neck, bile duct, brain, and stomach cancers; Hodgkin lymphoma, non-Hodgkin lymphoma, clear cell sarcoma, leukemia; and one unknown primary.

We found that airport runoff of jet fuel and deicing fluid had entered the Rocky River, which runs next to Building 500. However, jet fuel and deicing fluids are not known to cause cancer, and the river was not a source of drinking water for building occupants, who are supplied with city water. Much of the asbestos in Buildings 500 and 501 had been removed over the years, but some was still managed in place and posed no hazard to building occupants. We identified minor IEQ problems, such as water damage to ceiling tiles and walls, and in some cases poor maintenance of fan coil units, but these are not associated with the cancers that were diagnosed among employees of Buildings 500 and 501.

We found no evidence that the cancers reported are associated with work in Buildings 500 and 501 because the number and types of cancers do not appear unusual, the different types of cancers do not suggest a common exposure, no significant hazardous exposures were identified, and evidence leads to nonoccupational causes. Although we recommend no further investigation into the cancers reported in these buildings, employees may have concerns about their own risk for cancer. Therefore, management and the union should take this opportunity to encourage employees to learn about known cancer risk factors, measures they can take to reduce their risk for preventable cancers, and availability of cancer screening programs for certain types of cancer.

Keywords: NAICS 927110 (Space Research and Technology), indoor environmental quality, IEQ, asbestos, cancer, mold, water.

On October 11, 2007, NIOSH received a request for an HHE from the management of the NASA GRC, Cleveland, Ohio. The request was about ongoing employee and union concerns about a possible higher rate of cancer among current and former employees of Buildings 500 and 501. This was the second HHE request NIOSH received regarding this issue. The first request, received in 2004, was also submitted by management. In this first request 20 to 25 cases of cancer, primarily breast cancer, had been reported among employees. At that time we identified no hazardous exposures and closed the HHE [NIOSH 2004]. In this later request, NASA GRC management explained that cancer concerns had resurfaced. According to NASA GRC management, no identified cause for these cancers had been identified, but employees were concerned about potential exposure to jet fuel and deicing compounds from the nearby airport, asbestos in the buildings, water damage in the buildings, and general IEQ.

Facility Description

The NASA GRC consists of approximately 150 buildings and more than 500 special research and test facilities. More than 2,500 employees and contractors work at the 350-acre Cleveland location and the 6,400-acre Plum Brook, Ohio site. The NASA GRC mainly does propulsion research and is working on the module that will power the crew exploration vehicle scheduled to replace the space shuttle.

This evaluation focused on the employees in Buildings 500 and 501. Each structure is a three-story brick office building constructed in the early 1960s, and both are situated on the NASA GRC campus across the road from the Cleveland Hopkins International Airport. Building 500 has approximately 110,000 square feet of office space, and Building 501 has about 25,000 square feet; neither building has research labs. About 400 employees and contractors work in these two buildings.

The ventilation systems in Buildings 500 and 501 are similar, with most of the individual offices in both buildings heated and cooled by individual fan coil units placed along the exterior walls. In Building 501, the office suites on the partially below-ground garden level (the lowest level) are served by a forced-air HVAC system that has a rooftop outdoor air intake. According to NASA management, this system provided 100% outdoor air. Some offices

INTRODUCTION
(CONTINUED)

on the garden level of Building 501 had freestanding dehumidifiers (provided by NASA GRC and available at an employee's request). An HVAC mechanical room was also located on the garden level.

The larger spaces in Building 500, including the auditorium, draft room, dining room, and lobby, as well as most of the basement areas, are served by three forced-air HVAC systems. The HVAC mechanical room in Building 500 is in the basement, and the cooling tower is behind the building adjacent to the loading dock. The below-ground level outdoor air intakes for the three forced-air HVAC systems in Building 500 were not near the cooling tower, loading dock, or other potential contaminant sources and were clean of leaves and other debris. Restrooms in both buildings were directly vented outside through the roof by powered exhaust fans.

ASSESSMENT

We reviewed numerous reports provided by NASA GRC management concerning asbestos remediation in these buildings, responses to complaints from building occupants, and environmental sampling during the past 14 years. We evaluated surveys about cancer diagnoses from current and former employees in Buildings 500 and 501 that were provided to us by employees, LESA, and NASA management. Additionally, an anonymous list of employees with cancer was sent by a supervisor, and the NASA GRC human resources office provided a list of medical and regular retirements from the buildings during the past 5 years. We spoke with representatives from the Ohio Environmental Protection Agency regarding any past or current environmental contamination issues near Buildings 500 and 501.

After reviewing the environmental reports and evaluating the employee surveys, we performed a site visit on October 7–8, 2008. On October 7, we held an opening conference with representatives of management, LESA, the Ohio Department of Health, and the Ohio Environmental Protection Agency, then walked through the buildings, took measurements of IEQ comfort parameters, and looked for evidence of water damage, water incursion, visible mold, and other potential IEQ problems. Spot measurements were taken in both buildings for carbon dioxide, temperature, and relative humidity using a Q-TRAK™ Plus Indoor Air Quality Monitor, Model 8554 (TSI Incorporated, Shoreview, Minnesota). When conducting an IEQ survey, NIOSH investigators often measure ventilation and comfort indicators, such as carbon dioxide, temperature, and relative humidity to provide information relative to the functioning and control of HVAC systems. On October 8, we gave two presentations to employees regarding the findings of our evaluation of the potential cancer cluster, and then had a closing conference with representatives of management and LESA.

RESULTS

Building Surveys

Exposures of concern to the union and employees included environmental contamination of the Rocky River, which runs near the buildings, from airport runoff of jet fuel and deicing fluid. Cleveland Hopkins International Airport currently uses propylene glycol as its deicing agent, but used ethylene glycol in the past. Neither is known to be a carcinogen, and propylene glycol is a food and cosmetic additive that is generally recognized as safe by the Food and Drug Administration [ATSDR 2007a; ATSDR 2007b]. Commercial jet fuel is kerosene-based and also not known to be a carcinogen [Health Protection Agency 2006]. The Rocky River runs near Building 500, but is not a source of drinking water for building occupants, who are supplied with city water.

Another exposure of concern to NASA GRC employees is asbestos. Based on our review of previous asbestos remediation projects in these buildings, much of the asbestos in Buildings 500 and 501 has been removed over the years, but some asbestos is still managed in place. Although asbestos is known to cause lung cancer and mesothelioma, it has not been shown to cause the other types of cancer reported among Building 500 and 501 employees. Furthermore, because the remaining asbestos present in both buildings is being properly managed in place, exposures among office employees would be minimal.

Radon, which causes lung cancer, can be present in buildings. However, radon levels in Buildings 500 and 501 should not be a problem because the offices are well ventilated and are in counties with a low (less than 2 picoCuries/liter) predicted average indoor radon level [EPA 2008a]. Seven employees were reported to have had lung cancer, three of whom smoked and one who did not. Information about smoking was not available for the other three employees with lung cancer because the diagnoses were reported by others.

The carbon dioxide concentrations in the occupied spaces of both buildings were within 700 parts per million of the outdoor concentrations, suggesting that the ventilation was adequate [ANSI/ASHRAE 2007]. Temperature and relative humidity were within ASHRAE-recommended thermal comfort guidelines [ANSI/ASHRAE 2004].

During our walk-through survey, Building 500 employees in several offices on the upper floors mentioned instances of flooding from a damaged roof drain or leaks from windows or fan coil units. We observed no visible mold in these areas, and repairs to the roof drain, windows, or fan coil units had addressed these problems. Several offices in Building 501 showed evidence of previous water damage on ceilings and walls from water leaks from the fan coil units on the floor above. One garden-level room had a recent water leak that had resulted in visible wall and ceiling tile damage. One of the damaged ceiling tiles also appeared to have some mold growth. In another room on the second floor of Building 501 the carpet had been damaged by water, resulting in some mold growth. As a result of the water damage this office was not currently occupied. The NASA GRC health and safety office had collected air samples for mold, and access to the office was restricted until it was cleaned. The drains or drain tubes on some condensate drip pans in Building 501 were either completely or partially plugged. In one instance the drain tube was not properly connected to the drain. Several of the condensate drip pans were rusty.

The interiors of some of the fan coil units randomly selected for inspection in both buildings were clean and well maintained. However, the interiors of several other randomly selected fan coil units had visible dust inside the cabinet. Although the internal air filters on the fan coil units are changed yearly, several fan coil units had dust buildup that caused the filter to bend, permitting air to bypass the filter. In other fan coil units the air filter had been improperly installed or the fan shroud panel was missing screws, conditions that could affect the proper fit of the filters. The rubber foam attached to the air conditioning coil cover in some fan coil units was disintegrating, presumably from age.

In both buildings we observed metal ducting or pieces of cloth that had been placed over the supply vent on several fan coil units by employees working in the immediate area, presumably to redirect or reduce the airflow from these units. Employees had also placed extra fan coil unit filters over the supply vent to (according to employees) reduce particulates. In addition, access to the access panel of several fan coil units was restricted by furniture.

Housekeeping products used at the NASA GRC included Comet Cleanser, Zep® Disinfectant Cleaner, Zep Carpet Spot Remover, Simple Green® cleaner, Oxy-Force® cleaner, and antibacterial hand soap. Microfiber cloths, dust mops, and HEPA vacuums are used by the custodial staff. Carpets are cleaned with hot water (not steam). An integrated pest management approach is followed, resulting in a limited use of sprays and powders. For lawn care, herbicides, fungicides, and insecticides are applied as needed; fertilizers and weed control products are used approximately four times a year.

Employee Surveys

Because of the significant overlap between the sources of information about employees with cancer, duplicates were removed and people were contacted to confirm information (if possible). Of the 301 reports of people with cancer or other diagnoses, 23 were reported by persons other than the affected individual. Of these 301 current and former employees of Buildings 500 and 501, 63 reported having been diagnosed with cancer since 1985. Two people had two different primary cancers. Of the 63, five were diagnosed with cancer prior to working in these buildings and another eight were diagnosed within 5 years of beginning work in the buildings.

The employees diagnosed with cancer after beginning work in the buildings were spread throughout the buildings. Among employees of Buildings 500 and 501, 20 different types of cancer were diagnosed; the most common types were breast (17 cases), lung (7 cases), and prostate (4 cases).

DISCUSSION

Building Surveys

Overall, the IEQ of Buildings 500 and 501 was good during this evaluation. We saw evidence of previous water leaks and water damage in several offices in both buildings, which can lead to poor IEQ if not properly addressed. Plugged drain tubes or drains in condensate drip pans prevent condensate water from properly draining and may eventually result in water leaking from the fan coil units. Water damage in the buildings may not only affect the structural integrity of the buildings but may cause chemical emissions and foster microbial growth, such as mold or fungi. Ingestion of certain types of fungal toxins is known to cause specific cancers but there is no evidence of carcinogenicity from indoor environmental exposures.

The frequency with which fan coil units are inspected may be insufficient, based on our observations of dusty or improperly installed air filters, plugged or disconnected condensate drain tubes, rusty condensate drip pans, and dust on the interior of randomly selected fan coils. The use of cloth, air filters, or metal ducting over the supply vents of some fan coil units in both buildings suggests that airflow from these units may need to be adjusted to improve employee comfort.

The NASA GRC created the Clean Team in late 2005 to assess root causes for poor IEQ and to develop corrective actions. Representatives from three divisions at the NASA GRC (Logistics and Technical Information; Facilities; and Safety, Health, and Environmental) evaluate health complaints reported for the entire Center. The Clean Team has been involved in mold remediation, roof and masonry maintenance, janitorial services, interior painting, and carpet replacement. A few of the Clean Team's accomplishments include increasing the use of HEPA vacuums and "green" cleaning products by janitorial staff, switching to hot-water carpet cleaning (no detergents), and daily review of work requests relating to water leaks and other IEQ concerns. The Clean Team also has an extensive array of IEQ survey equipment, including photo-ionization detectors, moisture meters, thermal imaging cameras, particle counters, and direct-reading monitors for carbon dioxide, temperature, and relative humidity.

Employee Surveys

The most frequently diagnosed cancer types among the 301 current and former employees of Buildings 500 and 501 were breast, lung, and prostate, which are the three most common cancers in the United States. The other types of cancer diagnosed were melanoma, nonmelanoma skin cancer, colon, thyroid, bladder, pancreatic, cervical, uterine, head and neck, bile duct, brain, and stomach cancers; and Hodgkin lymphoma, non-Hodgkin lymphoma, clear cell sarcoma, leukemia; and one unknown primary. This section provides specific information on breast, lung, and prostate cancer.

Breast Cancer

An estimated 178,480 cases of invasive breast cancer were diagnosed in women in the United States in 2008, making it the most common cancer in women [American Cancer Society 2008a]. Although epidemiologic studies have identified some factors that appear to be related to increased risk for breast cancer, much remains unknown about the causes of breast cancer. Well-established risk factors include family history of breast cancer, biopsy-confirmed atypical hyperplasia, early menarche, late menopause, postmenopausal hormone replacement therapy, not having children or having the first child after age 30, alcohol consumption, overweight or obesity (especially after menopause), never breastfeeding a child, low physical activity levels, and higher levels of education and socioeconomic status [American Cancer Society 2008a]. Breast cancer is not known to be associated with environmental or occupational exposures other than high doses of ionizing radiation [Goldberg and Lebreche 1996; Wiederpass et al. 1999; Carmichael et al. 2003]. The risk is highest if exposure occurs during childhood and is negligible after age 40. Several studies have found teachers and other professional and managerial employees to have an increased risk for developing breast cancer [Rubin et al. 1993; King et al. 1994; Pollan and Gustavsson 1999; Bernstein et al. 2002; Snedeker 2006; MacArthur et al. 2007] but others have not [Coogan et al. 1996; Calle et al. 1998; Petralia et al. 1999]. No causative workplace exposures have been identified for these occupations, and it is postulated that the possible increase in risk is a result of nonoccupational risk factors such as parity, maternal age at first birth, contraceptive use, diet, and physical activity [Threlfell et al. 1985; Snedeker 2006; MacArthur et al. 2007]. Women with higher educational status are also more likely to have mammograms, thus increasing detection of breast cancer. A recent study compared the incidence of invasive breast cancer among women who were screened once between ages 50 and 64 to women screened three times between ages 50 and 64. Distribution of known risk factors was similar between the two groups, but the rate of invasive breast cancer was 22% lower in the group screened only once, suggesting that some breast cancers regress without treatment [Zahl et al. 2008].

Lung Cancer

Lung cancer is the most common cause of cancer death in both men and women. An estimated 215,020 new cases of lung cancer were diagnosed in 2008 [American Cancer Society 2008b]. The most significant risk factor for lung cancer is cigarette smoking, which accounts for 87% of cases in men and 85% in women [Miller 2000]. Radon is the most common cause of lung cancer in nonsmokers, and second most common cause of lung cancer overall, accounting for over 20,000 cases of lung cancer annually in the United States. Almost 3,000 of these cases occur in people who have never smoked [EPA 2008b]. Secondhand smoke is the third most common cause of lung cancer in the United States, with more than 3,000 cases annually [EPA 2008b; American Cancer Society 2008d]. Known occupational causes of lung cancer include asbestos, arsenic, chromium, nickel, cadmium, coke oven emissions, tars, and soot [American Cancer Society 2006].

Prostate Cancer

Prostate cancer is the most commonly diagnosed cancer among men in the United States, with 186,320 cases diagnosed in 2008 [American Cancer Society 2008b]. The main risk factor is increasing age; blacks are at higher risk. No occupational or environmental risk factors for prostate cancer are known. Exposure to certain substances, such as polycyclic aromatic hydrocarbons, pesticides, and cadmium have been suspected to increase the risk for prostate cancer, but study results conflict [Verougstraete et al. 2003; Boers et al. 2005; Sahmoun et al. 2005; Van Maele-Fabry et al. 2006; Huff et al. 2007; Mink et al. 2008].

Cancer Clusters

Because of the concerns among the NASA GRC employees about cancer, we believe it is helpful to review some general information about cancer and the approach we take in determining whether cancers have any relationship to the workplace. Cancer is a group of different diseases that have the same feature, the uncontrolled growth and spread of abnormal cells. Each different type of cancer may have its own set of causes. Cancer is common in the United States, accounting for one in every four deaths. Among adults, cancer is more frequent among men than women, and it is more frequent with increasing age.

Many factors play a role in the development of cancer. The importance of these factors varies for different types of cancer. Most cancers are caused by a combination of several factors. Some of the factors include (a) personal characteristics such as age, sex, and race; (b) family history of cancer; (c) diet; (d) personal habits such as cigarette smoking and alcohol consumption; (e) the presence of certain medical conditions; (f) exposure to cancer-causing agents in the environment; and (g) exposure to cancer-causing agents in the workplace. In many cases, these factors may act together or in sequence to cause cancer. Although some causes of some types of cancer are known, we do not know everything about the causes of cancer.

Cancers often appear to occur in clusters, which scientists define as an unusual concentration of cancer cases in a defined area or time [CDC 1990]. A cluster also occurs when the cancers are found among employees of a different age group or sex than is usual. The cases of cancer may have a common cause or may be the coincidental occurrence of unrelated causes. The number of cases may seem high, particularly among the small group of people who have something in common with the cases, such as working in the same building. It is common for the borders of the perceived cluster to be drawn around where the cases of cancer are located, instead of defining the population and geographic area first. This often leads to the inaccurate belief that the rate of cancer is high. Although the occurrence of a disease may be random, diseases often are not distributed randomly in the population, and clusters of disease may arise by chance alone [Metz and McGuinness 1997]. In many workplaces the number of cases is small. This makes detecting whether the cases have a common cause difficult, especially when no apparent cancer-causing exposures are present.

When cancer in a workplace is described, learning whether the type of cancer is a primary cancer or a metastasis (spread of the primary cancer into other organs) is important. Only primary cancers are used to investigate a cancer cluster. To assess whether the cancers among employees could be related to occupational exposures, we consider the number of cancer cases, the types of cancer, the likelihood of exposures to potential cancer-causing agents, and the timing of the diagnosis of cancer in relation to the exposure. These issues are discussed below in a series of questions that relate to the situation at the NASA GRC.

Do more NASA GRC employees in Buildings 500 and 501 have cancer than people who do not work in Buildings 500 and 501?

Because cancer is a common disease, cancer may be found among people at any workplace. In the United States, one in two men and one in three women will develop cancer over the course of their lifetimes. These numbers do not include basal or squamous cell skin cancers, which are very common (more than 1 million diagnosed annually), or any in-situ carcinomas other than bladder. (In-situ refers to cancer that has not yet spread beyond where it began; it is considered a precursor form of cancer.) If these were included, rates would be even higher. When several cases of cancer occur in a workplace they may be part of a true cluster when the number is greater than we expect compared to other groups of people similar in age, sex, and race. Disease or tumor rates, however, are highly variable in small populations and rarely match the overall rate for a larger area, such as the state, so that for any given time period some populations have rates above the overall rate and others have rates below the overall rate. So, even when a higher rate occurs, this may be completely consistent with the expected random variability. In addition, calculations like this make many assumptions that may not be appropriate for every workplace. Comparing rates without adjusting for age, sex, or other population characteristics assumes that such characteristics are the same in the workplace as in the larger population, which may not be true. However, general information on cancer rates can be useful for providing perspective on the cancers in your population. Therefore, even though comparing the cancer rate among Building 500 and 501 employees to a standard population is difficult, the numbers of cancers found among current and former Building 500 and 501 employees does not appear excessive.

Do Buildings 500 and 501 have an unusual distribution of types of cancer?

Twenty different types of cancer were diagnosed among employees of Buildings 500 and 501, but the most common types of cancer diagnosed were breast, lung, and prostate, the three most common cancers in the United States. The other types of cancer diagnosed were melanoma, nonmelanoma skin cancer, colon, thyroid, bladder, pancreatic, cervical, uterine, head and neck, bile duct, brain, and stomach cancers; Hodgkin lymphoma, non-Hodgkin lymphoma, clear cell sarcoma, leukemia; and one unknown primary.

Cancer clusters thought to be related to a workplace exposure usually consist of the same types of cancer. When several cases of the same type of cancer occur and that type is not common in the general population, it is more likely that an occupational exposure is involved. When the cluster consists of multiple types of cancer such as at the NASA GRC, without one type predominating, then an occupational cause of the cluster is less likely.

Is exposure to a specific chemical or physical agent known or suspected of causing cancer occurring in either Building 500 or 501?

We identified no chemical or physical agents based on our review of previous environmental reports or from our walk-through surveys of both buildings that would link potential workplace exposures to the reported cancers. In the scientific literature, the relationship between some agents and certain cancers has been well established. For other agents and cancers, the evidence is not definitive, but a suspicion exists. When a known or suspected cancer-causing agent is present and the types of cancer occurring have been linked with these exposures in other settings, we are more likely to make the connection between cancer and a workplace exposure. Neither of these criteria is met for the NASA GRC.

Has enough time passed since exposure began?

Five employees reported their cancer was diagnosed prior to working in Buildings 500 and 501, and another eight were diagnosed within 5 years of beginning work in the buildings. Latency periods (the time between first exposure to a cancer-causing agent and clinical recognition of the disease) vary by cancer type, but usually are a minimum of 10–12 years [Rugo 2004]. For example, it can take up to 30 years after exposure to asbestos for mesothelioma to develop. Because of this, past exposures are more relevant than current exposures as potential causes of cancers occurring in employees today.

CONCLUSIONS

We found no evidence that the cancers reported are associated with work in Buildings 500 and 501 for the following reasons: (a) the number and types of cancers do not appear unusual, (b) the different types of cancers do not suggest a common exposure, (c) no significant hazardous exposures were identified, and (d) evidence leads to nonoccupational causes.

The overall IEQ in Buildings 500 and 501 was good during our evaluation, and we identified no chemical or physical agents that would link potential workplace exposures to the reported cancers. However, we found evidence of previous water leaks and water damage in several offices in both buildings and poor maintenance of some fan coil units, which can lead to poor IEQ if not properly addressed.

RECOMMENDATIONS

We recommend no further investigation into the cancers reported in these two buildings. Although cancers among Building 500 and 501 employees are not likely due to exposures at work, employees may have concerns about their own risk for cancer. Therefore, management and the union should take this opportunity to encourage employees to learn about the following:

- Known cancer risk factors
- Measures to reduce individual risk for preventable cancers
- Availability of cancer screening programs for certain types of cancer

The American Cancer Society posts information about cancer on its website at www.cancer.org. For general information, click on "All about cancer" under "Patients, Family, & Friends." For information about a specific type of cancer, click on "Choose a cancer topic," select a type of cancer, then click "Go." Additionally, NIOSH posts information about occupational cancer and cancer cluster evaluations on its website at www.cdc.gov/niosh/topics/cancer.

Employees can take an active role in changing the personal risk factors associated with certain types of cancer. In fact, the American Cancer Society estimates that half of all cancer deaths in the United States were preventable [American Cancer Society 2008c]. In 2008, tobacco use alone caused an estimated 170,000

RECOMMENDATIONS
(CONTINUED)

cancer deaths. It is well known that tobacco use is the single largest preventable cause of disease and increases the risk of 14 types of cancer including lung, mouth, nasal cavity, larynx, pharynx, esophagus, stomach, liver, pancreas, kidney, bladder, uterine, cervix, and myeloid leukemia. High alcohol consumption, a diet low in fruits and vegetables, physical inactivity, overweight, and obesity are other modifiable personal risk factors that increase the risk of certain cancers. In fact, approximately one third of all cancer deaths in 2008 were related to poor nutrition, physical inactivity, and a high body mass index (a relationship between weight and height associated with body fat and health risk). Abundant scientific evidence shows that higher body mass index is associated with an increased risk of 15 types of cancer including esophagus, stomach, colorectal, liver, gallbladder, pancreas, prostate, kidney, non-Hodgkin lymphoma, multiple myeloma, leukemia, breast, uterus, cervix, and ovary.

Another substantial way for employees to prevent morbidity and mortality from cancer is to get cancer screening tests recommended for persons of their age and/or sex (e.g., colonoscopies for colon cancer screening, mammograms for breast cancer screening). Employees need to discuss available cancer screening programs with their primary care physicians. This can lead to earlier detection of cancers and earlier treatment, which may increase the chances of cancer remission or cure.

NASA GRC should improve maintenance of fan coil units in Buildings 500 and 501, including more frequent inspections to check the condensate drain pans, proper fitting of air filters, and general cleanliness of the fan coil cabinet interiors.

REFERENCES

ATSDR [2007a]. Toxicological profile for the ethylene glycol (*Draft for Public Comment*). Agency for Toxic Substances and Disease Registry, Atlanta, GA: U.S. Department of Health and Human Services.

ATSDR [2007b]. Case studies in environmental medicine: ethylene glycol and propylene glycol toxicity. Agency for Toxic Substances and Disease Registry, Atlanta, GA: U.S. Department of Health and Human Services. [www.atsdr.cdc.gov/csem/egpg/propylene_glycol.html]. Date accessed: December 5, 2008.

American Cancer Society [2006]. Occupation and cancer. Atlanta GA: American Cancer Society. [www.cancer.org/docroot/PRO/content/PRO_1_1x_Occupation_and_Cancer pdf. asp?sitearea=PRO]. Date accessed: November 19, 2008.

American Cancer Society [2008a]. Breast cancer facts and figures 2007–2008. Atlanta GA: American Cancer Society. [www.cancer.org/docroot/STT/stt_0_2007.asp?sitearea=STT&level=1]. Date accessed: November 19, 2008.

American Cancer Society [2008b]. Cancer facts & figures. Atlanta GA: American Cancer Society. [www.cancer.org/docroot/STT/content/STT_1x_Cancer_Facts_and_Figures_2008.asp?from=fast]. Date accessed: November 18, 2008.

American Cancer Society [2008c]. Cancer prevention and early detection facts & figures 2008. [www.cancer.org/docroot/STT/content/STT_1x_Cancer_Prevention__Early_Detection_Facts__Figures_2008 asp]. Date accessed: November 18, 2008.

American Cancer Society [2008d]. Prevention and early detection: secondhand smoke. Atlanta GA: American Cancer Society. [www.cancer.org/docroot/PED/content/PED_10_2X_Secondhand_Smoke-Clean_Indoor_Air.asp]. Date accessed: January 16, 2009.

ANSI/ASHRAE [2004]. Thermal environmental conditions for human occupancy. American National Standards Institute/ASHRAE standard 55-2004. Atlanta, GA: American Society for Heating, Refrigerating, and Air-Conditioning Engineers, Inc.

ANSI/ASHRAE [2007]. Ventilation for acceptable indoor air quality. American National Standards Institute/ASHRAE standard 62.1-2007. Atlanta, GA: American Society of Heating, Refrigerating, and Air-Conditioning Engineers, Inc.

Bernstein L, Allen M, Anton-Culver H, Deapen D, Horn-Ross PL, Peel D, Pinder R, Reynolds P, Sullivan-Halley J, West D, Wright W, Ziogas A, Ross RK [2002]. High breast cancer incidence rates among California teachers: results from the California Teachers Study (United States). Cancer Causes Control 13(7):625–635.

Boers D, Zeegers MPA, Swaen GM, Kant I, van den Brandt PA [2005]. The influence of occupational exposure to pesticides, polycyclic aromatic hydrocarbons, diesel exhaust, metal dust, metal

REFERENCES
(CONTINUED)

fumes, and mineral oil on prostate cancer: a prospective cohort study. Occup Environ Med 62(8):531–537.

Calle EE, Murphy TK, Rodriguez C, Thun MJ, Heath CW [1998]. Occupation and breast cancer mortality in a prospective cohort of U.S. women. Am J Epidemiol 148(2):191–197.

Carmichael A, Sami AS, Dixon JM [2003]. Breast cancer risk among the survivors of atomic bomb and patients exposed to therapeutic ionizing radiation. Eur J Surg Oncol 29(5):475–479.

CDC (Centers for Disease Control and Prevention) [1990]. Guidelines for investigating clusters of health events. MMWR 39(11).

Coogan PF, Clapp RW, Newcomb PA, Mittendorf R, Bogdan G, Baron JA, Longnecker MP [1996]. Variation in female breast cancer risk by occupation. Am J Ind Med 30(4):430–437.

EPA [2008a]. Environmental Protection Agency map of radon zones. [www.epa.gov/radon/zonemap.html]. Date accessed: December 3, 2008.

EPA [2008b]. Radon health risks. [www.epa.gov/radon/healthrisks.html]. Date accessed: January 16, 2009.

Goldberg MS, Labreche F [1996]. Occupational risk factors for female breast cancer: a review. Occup Environ Med 53(3):145–156.

Health Protection Agency [2006]. Compendium of chemical hazards: kerosene (fuel oil). [www.who int/ipcs/emergencies/kerosene.pdf]. Date accessed: December 5, 2008.

Huff J, Lunn RM, Waalkes MP, Tomatis L, Infante PF [2007]. Cadmium-induced cancers in animals and in humans. Int J Occup Environ Health 13(2):202–212.

King AS, Threlfall WJ, Band PR, Gallagher RP [1994]. Mortality among female registered nurses and school teachers in British Columbia. Am J Ind Med 26(1):125–132.

MacArthur AC, Le ND, Abanto ZU, Gallagher RP [2007]. Occupational female breast and reproductive cancer mortality in British Columbia, Canada, 1950-94. Occup Med 57(4):246–253.

REFERENCES
(CONTINUED)

Metz LM, McGuinness S [1997]. Responding to reported clusters of common diseases: the case of multiple sclerosis. Can J Public Health 88(4):277–279.

Miller YE [2000]. Pulmonary neoplasms. In: Goldman L, Bennett JC, eds. Cecil textbook of medicine. 21st rev. ed. Philadelphia, PA: WB Saunders Co, pp. 449–455.

Mink PJ, Adami H-O, Trichopoulos D, Britton NL, Mandel JS [2008]. Pesticides and prostate cancer: a review of epidemiologic studies with specific agricultural exposure information. Europ J Cancer Prev 17(2):97–110.

NIOSH [2004]. Health hazard evaluation closeout letter. NASA Glenn Research Center, Cleveland, OH. Cincinnati, OH: U.S. Department of Health and Human Services, Centers for Disease Control and Prevention, National Institute for Occupational Safety and Health, NIOSH HETA No. 2004-0299.

Petralia SA, Vena JE, Freudenehim JL, Michalek A, Goldberg MS, Blair A, Brasure J, Graham S [1999]. Risk of premenopausal breast cancer and patterns of established breast cancer risk factors among teachers and nurses. Am J Ind Med 35(1):137–141.

Pollan M, Gustavsson P [1999]. High-risk occupations for breast cancer in Swedish female working populations. Am J Public Health 89(6):875–881.

Rubin CH, Burnett CA, Halperin WE, Seligman PJ [1993]. Occupation as a risk identifier for breast cancer. Am J Public Health 83(9):1311–1315.

Rugo HS [2004]. Occupational cancer. In: La Dou J, ed. Current occupational and environmental medicine. 3rd rev. ed. New York: McGraw Hill Companies, Inc., pp. 229–267.

Sahmoun AE, Case LD, Jackson SA, Schwartz GG [2005]. Cadmium and prostate cancer: a critical epidemiologic analysis. Cancer Invest 23(3):256–263.

Snedeker SM [2006]. Chemical exposures in the workplace: effect on breast cancer risk among women. AAOHN J 54(6):270–279.

References
(continued)

Threlfall WJ, Gallagher RP, Spinelli JJ, Band P [1985]. Reproductive variables as possible confounders in occupational studies of breast and ovarian cancer in females. J Occup Environ Med 27(6):448–450.

Van Maele-Fabry G, Libotte V, Willems J, Lison D [2006]. Review and meta-analysis of risk estimates for prostate cancer in pesticide manufacturing workers. Cancer Causes Control 17(4):353–373.

Verougstraete V, Lison D, Hotz P [2003]. Cadmium, lung and prostate cancer: a systematic review of recent epidemiological data. J Toxicol Environ Health 6(3):227–255.

Weiderpass E, Pukkala E, Kauppinen T, Mutanen P, Paakkulainen H, Vasama-Neuvonen K, Boffetta P, Partanen T [1999]. Breast cancer and occupational exposures in women in Finland. Am J Ind Med 36(1):48–53.

Zahl P-H, Maehlen J, Welch HG [2008]. The natural history of invasive breast cancers detected by screening mammography. Arch Int Med 168(21):2311–2316.

This page intentionally left blank

ACKNOWLEDGMENTS AND AVAILABILITY OF REPORT

The Hazard Evaluations and Technical Assistance Branch (HETAB) of the National Institute for Occupational Safety and Health (NIOSH) conducts field investigations of possible health hazards in the workplace. These investigations are conducted under the authority of Section 20(a)(6) of the Occupational Safety and Health Administration (OSHA) Act of 1970, 29 U.S.C. 669(a)(6) which authorizes the Secretary of Health and Human Services, following a written request from any employer or authorized representative of employees, to determine whether any substance normally found in the place of employment has potentially toxic effects in such concentrations as used or found. HETAB also provides, upon request, technical and consultative assistance to federal, state, and local agencies; labor; industry; and other groups or individuals to control occupational health hazards and to prevent related trauma and disease.

The findings and conclusions in this report are those of the authors and do not necessarily represent the views of NIOSH. Mention of any company or product does not constitute endorsement by NIOSH. In addition, citations to websites external to NIOSH do not constitute NIOSH endorsement of the sponsoring organization or their programs or products. Furthermore, NIOSH is not responsible for the content of these websites. All Web addresses referenced in this document were accessible as of the publication date.

This report was prepared by Elena Page, Gregory Burr, and Scott Brueck of HETAB, Division of Surveillance, Hazard Evaluations and Field Studies (DSHEFS). Medical field assistance was provided by Marie DePerio and Tony Almazan of DSHEFS. Technical support was provided by Robert Indian of the Ohio Department of Health and Nancy Zikmanis of the Ohio Environmental Protection Agency. Health communication assistance was provided by Stefanie Evans. Editorial assistance was provided by Ellen Galloway. Desktop publishing was performed by Robin Smith.

Copies of this report have been sent to employee and management representatives at the NASA Glenn Research Center, the Lewis Engineers and Scientists Association, and the OSHA Regional Office. This report is not copyrighted and may be freely reproduced. The report may be viewed and printed from www.cdc.gov/niosh/hhe. Copies may be purchased from the National Technical Information Service at 5825 Port Royal Road, Springfield, Virginia 22161.

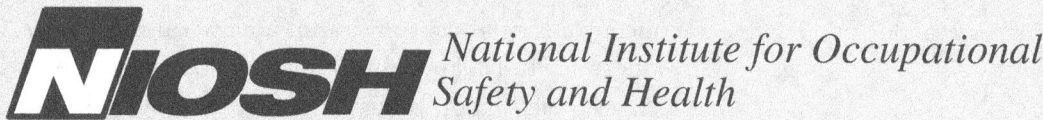 *National Institute for Occupational Safety and Health*

Delivering on the Nation's promise: Safety and health at work for all people through research and prevention.

To receive NIOSH documents or information about occupational safety and health topics, contact NIOSH at:

1-800-CDC-INFO (1-800-232-4636)

TTY: 1-888-232-6348

E-mail: cdcinfo@cdc.gov

or visit the NIOSH web site at: **www.cdc.gov/niosh.**

For a monthly update on news at NIOSH, subscribe to NIOSH eNews by visiting **www.cdc.gov/niosh/eNews.**

SAFER • HEALTHIER • PEOPLE™